Monitoring Blood Sugar - for Women

© Copyright 2016, by

Ahl Kayn Publications

Spring Valley, New York

ISBN-13: 978-1539022312
ISBN-10: 1539022315
First Printing - 2016

Manufactured in the United States of America

Monitoring Blood Sugar - for Women

The purpose of this Blood Sugar Log is threefold:

- Know how your blood sugar varies over time after eating
- Pinpoint what foods spike your blood sugar
- Pinpoint how much food causes a spike in your blood sugar

This log works for whatever monitoring schedule you choose, whether it be every meal or whenever it is convenient to take your reading.

At some point in your logging you will begin to see patterns, and that will allow you to adjust the kinds of foods and the specific portion size changes to have the greatest reduction in blood sugar spiking with the least inconvenience

Date:		Reading Before	Reading 1 hr After	Reading 2 hrs After	Reading 4 hrs After
Which Meal:					
Time Start:					
Time End:					
What I Ate and How Much					
Comments :					

Date:		Reading Before	Reading 1 hr After	Reading 2 hrs After	Reading 4 hrs After
Which Meal:					
Time Start:					
Time End:					
What I Ate and How Much					
Comments :					

Date:		Reading Before	Reading 1 hr After	Reading 2 hrs After	Reading 4 hrs After
Which Meal:					
Time Start:					
Time End:					
What I Ate and How Much					
Comments :					

Date:		Reading Before	Reading 1 hr After	Reading 2 hrs After	Reading 4 hrs After
Which Meal:					
Time Start:					
Time End:					
What I Ate and How Much					
Comments :					

Date:		Reading Before	Reading 1 hr After	Reading 2 hrs After	Reading 4 hrs After
Which Meal:					
Time Start:					
Time End:					
What I Ate and How Much					
Comments :					

Date:		Reading Before	Reading 1 hr After	Reading 2 hrs After	Reading 4 hrs After
Which Meal:					
Time Start:					
Time End:					
What I Ate and How Much					
Comments :					

Date:		Reading Before	Reading 1 hr After	Reading 2 hrs After	Reading 4 hrs After
Which Meal:					
Time Start:					
Time End:					
What I Ate and How Much					
Comments :					

Date:		Reading Before	Reading 1 hr After	Reading 2 hrs After	Reading 4 hrs After
Which Meal:					
Time Start:					
Time End:					
What I Ate and How Much					
Comments :					

Date:		Reading Before	Reading 1 hr After	Reading 2 hrs After	Reading 4 hrs After
Which Meal:					
Time Start:					
Time End:					
What I Ate and How Much					
Comments :					

Date:		Reading Before	Reading 1 hr After	Reading 2 hrs After	Reading 4 hrs After
Which Meal:					
Time Start:					
Time End:					
What I Ate and How Much					
Comments :					

Date:		Reading Before	Reading 1 hr After	Reading 2 hrs After	Reading 4 hrs After
Which Meal:					
Time Start:					
Time End:					
What I Ate and How Much					
Comments :					

Date:		Reading Before	Reading 1 hr After	Reading 2 hrs After	Reading 4 hrs After
Which Meal:					
Time Start:					
Time End:					
What I Ate and How Much					
Comments :					

Date:		Reading Before	Reading 1 hr After	Reading 2 hrs After	Reading 4 hrs After
Which Meal:					
Time Start:					
Time End:					
What I Ate and How Much					
Comments :					

Date:		Reading Before	Reading 1 hr After	Reading 2 hrs After	Reading 4 hrs After
Which Meal:					
Time Start:					
Time End:					
What I Ate and How Much					
Comments :					

Date:		Reading Before	Reading 1 hr After	Reading 2 hrs After	Reading 4 hrs After
Which Meal:					
Time Start:					
Time End:					
What I Ate and How Much					
Comments :					

Date:		Reading Before	Reading 1 hr After	Reading 2 hrs After	Reading 4 hrs After
Which Meal:					
Time Start:					
Time End:					
What I Ate and How Much					
Comments :					

Date:		Reading Before	Reading 1 hr After	Reading 2 hrs After	Reading 4 hrs After
Which Meal:					
Time Start:					
Time End:					
What I Ate and How Much					
Comments :					

Date:		Reading Before	Reading 1 hr After	Reading 2 hrs After	Reading 4 hrs After
Which Meal:					
Time Start:					
Time End:					
What I Ate and How Much					
Comments :					

Date:		Reading Before	Reading 1 hr After	Reading 2 hrs After	Reading 4 hrs After
Which Meal:					
Time Start:					
Time End:					
What I Ate and How Much					
Comments :					

Date:		Reading Before	Reading 1 hr After	Reading 2 hrs After	Reading 4 hrs After
Which Meal:					
Time Start:					
Time End:					
What I Ate and How Much					
Comments :					

Date:		Reading Before	Reading 1 hr After	Reading 2 hrs After	Reading 4 hrs After
Which Meal:					
Time Start:					
Time End:					
What I Ate and How Much					
Comments :					

Date:		Reading Before	Reading 1 hr After	Reading 2 hrs After	Reading 4 hrs After
Which Meal:					
Time Start:					
Time End:					
What I Ate and How Much					
Comments :					

Date:		Reading Before	Reading 1 hr After	Reading 2 hrs After	Reading 4 hrs After
Which Meal:					
Time Start:					
Time End:					
What I Ate and How Much					
Comments :					

Date:		Reading Before	Reading 1 hr After	Reading 2 hrs After	Reading 4 hrs After
Which Meal:					
Time Start:					
Time End:					
What I Ate and How Much					
Comments :					

Date:		Reading Before	Reading 1 hr After	Reading 2 hrs After	Reading 4 hrs After
Which Meal:					
Time Start:					
Time End:					
What I Ate and How Much					
Comments :					

Date:		Reading Before	Reading 1 hr After	Reading 2 hrs After	Reading 4 hrs After
Which Meal:					
Time Start:					
Time End:					
What I Ate and How Much					
Comments :					

Date:		Reading Before	Reading 1 hr After	Reading 2 hrs After	Reading 4 hrs After
Which Meal:					
Time Start:					
Time End:					
What I Ate and How Much					
Comments :					

Date:		Reading Before	Reading 1 hr After	Reading 2 hrs After	Reading 4 hrs After
Which Meal:					
Time Start:					
Time End:					
What I Ate and How Much					
Comments :					

Date:		Reading Before	Reading 1 hr After	Reading 2 hrs After	Reading 4 hrs After
Which Meal:					
Time Start:					
Time End:					
What I Ate and How Much					
Comments :					

Date:		Reading Before	Reading 1 hr After	Reading 2 hrs After	Reading 4 hrs After
Which Meal:					
Time Start:					
Time End:					
What I Ate and How Much					
Comments :					

Date:		Reading Before	Reading 1 hr After	Reading 2 hrs After	Reading 4 hrs After
Which Meal:					
Time Start:					
Time End:					
What I Ate and How Much					
Comments:					

Date:		Reading Before	Reading 1 hr After	Reading 2 hrs After	Reading 4 hrs After
Which Meal:					
Time Start:					
Time End:					
What I Ate and How Much					
Comments:					

Date:		Reading Before	Reading 1 hr After	Reading 2 hrs After	Reading 4 hrs After
Which Meal:					
Time Start:					
Time End:					
What I Ate and How Much					
Comments:					

Date:		Reading Before	Reading 1 hr After	Reading 2 hrs After	Reading 4 hrs After
Which Meal:					
Time Start:					
Time End					
What I Ate and How Much					
Comments :					

Date:		Reading Before	Reading 1 hr After	Reading 2 hrs After	Reading 4 hrs After
Which Meal:					
Time Start:					
Time End:					
What I Ate and How Much					
Comments :					

Date:		Reading Before	Reading 1 hr After	Reading 2 hrs After	Reading 4 hrs After
Which Meal:					
Time Start:					
Time End:					
What I Ate and How Much					
Comments :					

Date:		Reading Before	Reading 1 hr After	Reading 2 hrs After	Reading 4 hrs After
Which Meal:					
Time Start:					
Time End:					
What I Ate and How Much					
Comments :					

Date:		Reading Before	Reading 1 hr After	Reading 2 hrs After	Reading 4 hrs After
Which Meal:					
Time Start:					
Time End:					
What I Ate and How Much					
Comments :					

Date:		Reading Before	Reading 1 hr After	Reading 2 hrs After	Reading 4 hrs After
Which Meal:					
Time Start:					
Time End:					
What I Ate and How Much					
Comments :					

		Reading Before	Reading 1 hr After	Reading 2 hrs After	Reading 4 hrs After
Date:					
Which Meal:					
Time Start:					
Time End:					
What I Ate and How Much					
Comments :					

		Reading Before	Reading 1 hr After	Reading 2 hrs After	Reading 4 hrs After
Date:					
Which Meal:					
Time Start:					
Time End:					
What I Ate and How Much					
Comments :					

		Reading Before	Reading 1 hr After	Reading 2 hrs After	Reading 4 hrs After
Date:					
Which Meal:					
Time Start:					
Time End:					
What I Ate and How Much					
Comments :					

Date:		Reading Before	Reading 1 hr After	Reading 2 hrs After	Reading 4 hrs After
Which Meal:					
Time Start:					
Time End:					
What I Ate and How Much					
Comments :					

Date:		Reading Before	Reading 1 hr After	Reading 2 hrs After	Reading 4 hrs After
Which Meal:					
Time Start:					
Time End:					
What I Ate and How Much					
Comments :					

Date:		Reading Before	Reading 1 hr After	Reading 2 hrs After	Reading 4 hrs After
Which Meal:					
Time Start:					
Time End:					
What I Ate and How Much					
Comments :					

		Reading Before	Reading 1 hr After	Reading 2 hrs After	Reading 4 hrs After
Date:					
Which Meal:					
Time Start:					
Time End:					
What I Ate and How Much					
Comments :					

		Reading Before	Reading 1 hr After	Reading 2 hrs After	Reading 4 hrs After
Date:					
Which Meal:					
Time Start:					
Time End:					
What I Ate and How Much					
Comments :					

		Reading Before	Reading 1 hr After	Reading 2 hrs After	Reading 4 hrs After
Date:					
Which Meal:					
Time Start:					
Time End:					
What I Ate and How Much					
Comments :					

Date:		Reading Before	Reading 1 hr After	Reading 2 hrs After	Reading 4 hrs After
Which Meal:					
Time Start:					
Time End:					
What I Ate and How Much					
Comments :					

Date:		Reading Before	Reading 1 hr After	Reading 2 hrs After	Reading 4 hrs After
Which Meal:					
Time Start:					
Time End:					
What I Ate and How Much					
Comments :					

Date:		Reading Before	Reading 1 hr After	Reading 2 hrs After	Reading 4 hrs After
Which Meal:					
Time Start:					
Time End:					
What I Ate and How Much					
Comments :					

Date:		Reading Before	Reading 1 hr After	Reading 2 hrs After	Reading 4 hrs After
Which Meal:					
Time Start:					
Time End.					
What I Ate and How Much					
Comments :					

Date:		Reading Before	Reading 1 hr After	Reading 2 hrs After	Reading 4 hrs After
Which Meal:					
Time Start:					
Time End:					
What I Ate and How Much					
Comments :					

Date:		Reading Before	Reading 1 hr After	Reading 2 hrs After	Reading 4 hrs After
Which Meal:					
Time Start:					
Time End:					
What I Ate and How Much					
Comments :					

Date:		Reading Before	Reading 1 hr After	Reading 2 hrs After	Reading 4 hrs After
Which Meal:					
Time Start:					
Time End:					
What I Ate and How Much					
Comments:					

Date:		Reading Before	Reading 1 hr After	Reading 2 hrs After	Reading 4 hrs After
Which Meal:					
Time Start:					
Time End:					
What I Ate and How Much					
Comments:					

Date:		Reading Before	Reading 1 hr After	Reading 2 hrs After	Reading 4 hrs After
Which Meal:					
Time Start:					
Time End:					
What I Ate and How Much					
Comments:					

Date:		Reading Before	Reading 1 hr After	Reading 2 hrs After	Reading 4 hrs After
Which Meal:					
Time Start:					
Time End:					
What I Ate and How Much					
Comments :					

Date:		Reading Before	Reading 1 hr After	Reading 2 hrs After	Reading 4 hrs After
Which Meal:					
Time Start:					
Time End:					
What I Ate and How Much					
Comments :					

Date:		Reading Before	Reading 1 hr After	Reading 2 hrs After	Reading 4 hrs After
Which Meal:					
Time Start:					
Time End:					
What I Ate and How Much					
Comments :					

Date:		Reading Before	Reading 1 hr After	Reading 2 hrs After	Reading 4 hrs After
Which Meal:					
Time Start:					
Time End:					
What I Ate and How Much					
Comments :					

Date:		Reading Before	Reading 1 hr After	Reading 2 hrs After	Reading 4 hrs After
Which Meal:					
Time Start:					
Time End:					
What I Ate and How Much					
Comments :					

Date:		Reading Before	Reading 1 hr After	Reading 2 hrs After	Reading 4 hrs After
Which Meal:					
Time Start:					
Time End:					
What I Ate and How Much					
Comments :					

Date:		Reading Before	Reading 1 hr After	Reading 2 hrs After	Reading 4 hrs After
Which Meal:					
Time Start:					
Time End:					
What I Ate and How Much					
Comments :					

Date:		Reading Before	Reading 1 hr After	Reading 2 hrs After	Reading 4 hrs After
Which Meal:					
Time Start:					
Time End:					
What I Ate and How Much					
Comments :					

Date:		Reading Before	Reading 1 hr After	Reading 2 hrs After	Reading 4 hrs After
Which Meal:					
Time Start:					
Time End:					
What I Ate and How Much					
Comments :					

Date:		Reading Before	Reading 1 hr After	Reading 2 hrs After	Reading 4 hrs After
Which Meal:					
Time Start:					
Time End:					
What I Ate and How Much					
Comments :					

Date:		Reading Before	Reading 1 hr After	Reading 2 hrs After	Reading 4 hrs After
Which Meal:					
Time Start:					
Time End:					
What I Ate and How Much					
Comments :					

Date:		Reading Before	Reading 1 hr After	Reading 2 hrs After	Reading 4 hrs After
Which Meal:					
Time Start:					
Time End:					
What I Ate and How Much					
Comments :					

Date:		Reading Before	Reading 1 hr After	Reading 2 hrs After	Reading 4 hrs After
Which Meal:					
Time Start:					
Time End:					
What I Ate and How Much					
Comments :					

Date:		Reading Before	Reading 1 hr After	Reading 2 hrs After	Reading 4 hrs After
Which Meal:					
Time Start:					
Time End:					
What I Ate and How Much					
Comments :					

Date:		Reading Before	Reading 1 hr After	Reading 2 hrs After	Reading 4 hrs After
Which Meal:					
Time Start:					
Time End:					
What I Ate and How Much					
Comments :					

Date:		Reading Before	Reading 1 hr After	Reading 2 hrs After	Reading 4 hrs After
Which Meal:					
Time Start:					
Time End:					
What I Ate and How Much					
Comments :					

Date:		Reading Before	Reading 1 hr After	Reading 2 hrs After	Reading 4 hrs After
Which Meal:					
Time Start:					
Time End:					
What I Ate and How Much					
Comments :					

Date:		Reading Before	Reading 1 hr After	Reading 2 hrs After	Reading 4 hrs After
Which Meal:					
Time Start:					
Time End:					
What I Ate and How Much					
Comments :					

Date:		Reading Before	Reading 1 hr After	Reading 2 hrs After	Reading 4 hrs After
Which Meal:					
Time Start:					
Time End:					
What I Ate and How Much					
Comments :					

Date:		Reading Before	Reading 1 hr After	Reading 2 hrs After	Reading 4 hrs After
Which Meal:					
Time Start:					
Time End:					
What I Ate and How Much					
Comments :					

Date:		Reading Before	Reading 1 hr After	Reading 2 hrs After	Reading 4 hrs After
Which Meal:					
Time Start:					
Time End:					
What I Ate and How Much					
Comments :					

Date:		Reading Before	Reading 1 hr After	Reading 2 hrs After	Reading 4 hrs After
Which Meal:					
Time Start:					
Time End:					
What I Ate and How Much					
Comments:					

Date:		Reading Before	Reading 1 hr After	Reading 2 hrs After	Reading 4 hrs After
Which Meal:					
Time Start:					
Time End:					
What I Ate and How Much					
Comments:					

Date:		Reading Before	Reading 1 hr After	Reading 2 hrs After	Reading 4 hrs After
Which Meal:					
Time Start:					
Time End:					
What I Ate and How Much					
Comments:					

		Reading Before	Reading 1 hr After	Reading 2 hrs After	Reading 4 hrs After
Date:					
Which Meal:					
Time Start:					
Time End:					
What I Ate and How Much					
Comments:					

		Reading Before	Reading 1 hr After	Reading 2 hrs After	Reading 4 hrs After
Date:					
Which Meal:					
Time Start:					
Time End:					
What I Ate and How Much					
Comments:					

		Reading Before	Reading 1 hr After	Reading 2 hrs After	Reading 4 hrs After
Date:					
Which Meal:					
Time Start:					
Time End:					
What I Ate and How Much					
Comments:					

Date:		Reading Before	Reading 1 hr After	Reading 2 hrs After	Reading 4 hrs After
Which Meal:					
Time Start:					
Time End:					
What I Ate and How Much					
Comments :					

Date:		Reading Before	Reading 1 hr After	Reading 2 hrs After	Reading 4 hrs After
Which Meal:					
Time Start:					
Time End:					
What I Ate and How Much					
Comments :					

Date:		Reading Before	Reading 1 hr After	Reading 2 hrs After	Reading 4 hrs After
Which Meal:					
Time Start:					
Time End:					
What I Ate and How Much					
Comments :					

Date:		Reading Before	Reading 1 hr After	Reading 2 hrs After	Reading 4 hrs After
Which Meal:					
Time Start:					
Time End:					
What I Ate and How Much					
Comments :					

Date:		Reading Before	Reading 1 hr After	Reading 2 hrs After	Reading 4 hrs After
Which Meal:					
Time Start:					
Time End:					
What I Ate and How Much					
Comments :					

Date:		Reading Before	Reading 1 hr After	Reading 2 hrs After	Reading 4 hrs After
Which Meal:					
Time Start:					
Time End:					
What I Ate and How Much					
Comments :					

Date:		Reading Before	Reading 1 hr After	Reading 2 hrs After	Reading 4 hrs After
Which Meal:					
Time Start:					
Time End:					
What I Ate and How Much					
Comments :					

Date:		Reading Before	Reading 1 hr After	Reading 2 hrs After	Reading 4 hrs After
Which Meal:					
Time Start:					
Time End:					
What I Ate and How Much					
Comments :					

Date:		Reading Before	Reading 1 hr After	Reading 2 hrs After	Reading 4 hrs After
Which Meal:					
Time Start:					
Time End:					
What I Ate and How Much					
Comments :					

Date:		Reading Before	Reading 1 hr After	Reading 2 hrs After	Reading 4 hrs After
Which Meal:					
Time Start:					
Time End:					
What I Ate and How Much					
Comments:					

Date:		Reading Before	Reading 1 hr After	Reading 2 hrs After	Reading 4 hrs After
Which Meal:					
Time Start:					
Time End:					
What I Ate and How Much					
Comments:					

Date:		Reading Before	Reading 1 hr After	Reading 2 hrs After	Reading 4 hrs After
Which Meal:					
Time Start:					
Time End:					
What I Ate and How Much					
Comments:					

BOOKS BY Irwin Tyler (Yirmi Tyler)

UNDERSTANDING QUANTUM - Volume 1
>   The Universe is Made Up of "Stuff"
UNDERSTANDING QUANTUM - Volume 2
>   The Universe Doesn't Make Any Sense
UNDERSTANDING QUANTUM - Volume 3
>   The Theory of Everything
POINTS OF HEALTH
>   The Effectiveness and Safety of Acupuncture and Acupressure
WHY ACUPUNCTURE? - When Conventional Medicine Isn't Working As You
Hoped
WHY ACUPRESSURE? - When Conventional Medicine Isn't Working As You
Hoped
WHY CHIROPRACTIC? - When Conventional Medicine Isn't Working As You
Hoped
WHY HOMEOPATHY? - When Conventional Medicine Isn't Working As You
Hoped
THE DIET CHOICE PROGRAM - Beat the Cravings and Enjoy Your Dinner
SO MANY GATES TO THE CITY... A GUIDE FOR THE MODERN PERPLEXE
>   A Book About Jewish Belief and Understanding, and Making Some Sense
>   Of It
TARGUM AMERICANA - BERESHIT / GENESIS
COLLECTING PAPER MONEY WITH CONFIDENCE
GRADING COINS WITH CONFIDENCE

All are available at:
    AMAZON.COM
Selected titles available at:
    LULU.COM
    CREATESPACE.COM
    AHL KAYN PUBLICATIONS WEB SITE